STREETWISE GUIDE
CHINESE HERBAL
MEDICINE

Wong Kang-Ying • Martha Dahlen

Wokman Press

Photographs: Andreas Hunnemeyer
Designed and printed by:
Communication Art Design & Printing Ltd.
19/F, China Hong Kong Tower
8-12 Hennessy Road
Wanchai, Hong Kong

Published by Wokman Press

ISBN 962-7316-02-4

T ABLE OF CONTENTS

This guide introduces Chinese herbal medicine as it is practiced today. Its purpose is to enable the visitor to a Chinese herb shop to know what is happening, to understand how the herbs fit into the greater context of the Chinese medical system, and to identify some of the most common herbs. At the end are a few recipes which the interested reader may try. This small book does not seek to teach—nor even to encourage—the casual reader to prescribe herbs for his ills. Indeed, we hope our explanations will discourage such self-prescribing as they build respect for the complex system of which medicinal herbs are a part.

In this vein, then, the initial chapters focus on Chinese medicine: its history, theory, principles, and practice. While comparable to its Western counterpart in being firmly grounded in rational principles, Chinese medicine differs radically in its fundamental concepts. This difference is conspicuous in the practical aspects of diagnosis and the prescription of medicines.

The last chapter of this section describes the mechanics of using Chinese medicine. It begins with consulting the doctor, continues with how the prescription is filled at the medicine shop, and ends with how the prescriptions are brewed to make the tea which is, finally, consumed.

The next, longest section comprises descriptions of 60 of the most commonly used herbs. "Herb", used here in the generic sense, refers to everything in the materia medica and includes minerals and animal matter as well as plant material. These descriptions are illustrated with photographs of the items as they appear in the shops.

Ginseng, probably the most famous of Chinese medicinal herbs in the West, is the subject of one chapter. Volumes could—and have—been written on its history, traditional uses, therapeutic value, and various forms. Notes here merely skim the surface and end with some practical advice on purchase and use.

The final chapters offer recipes for traditional tonic soups and for simple teas and drinks which can be prepared from some of the herbs described and which are mild enough to be suitable for anyone.

We hope our explanations, photographs and notes will not only satisfy curiosity but also stimulate interest and instill respect for one of the world's oldest institutions—Chinese herbal medicine.

身 體 健 康

Wong Kang-Ying 黃鏡凝
Martha Dahlen

History Of
Chinese Medicine

The traditional medical system of China has been in use for more than 3,000 years. Explicated, refined and corroborated in more than 5,000 medical works still extant, it is documented better than that of any other civilization. The earliest medical records are those of oracle bones and tortoise shells. These indicate that, by 1,000 BC, China had a medical administration within the government as well as the precursor of a system for examining and qualifying doctors. The profession then comprised four fields: nutrition, surgery, internal medicine, and veterinary medicine.

By the eighth century BC the fundamental principles of traditional Chinese medicine ("TCM" in its modern abbreviation) had been formulated. The Yellow Emperor's Canon of Internal Medicine (Huang Di Nei Jing, circa 722 B.C.), is the earliest recorded treatise in this field and it is still revered and studied as the ultimate theoretical reference for TCM.

Interestingly, while the principles of TCM focus on subtle energy circulation (and this is perhaps its most publicized divergence from Western medicine), the Chinese also knew much of anatomy. The Yellow Emperor's Canon records the length of human skeletons and blood vessels, and the position, shape, size and weights of internal organs. Many of these measurements are close to those of today. That the blood constantly circulates was stated in the Canon, which also dealt with the relationship of the movement of the aorta, breathing and the pulse rate.

The earliest book on pharmacology was Shen Nong's Canon on Materia Medica (Shen Nong Ben Cao Jing), published in the first century AD. The foundation of herbal medicine, however, is considered to be Li Shizhen's classic Compendium of Materia Medica (Ben Cao Gang Mu) published in the 16th century. It records names and descriptions of some 1800 herbs with more than 1000 line drawings. Many if not most of these substances are still being used today, and increasing numbers are finding their way into the Western pharmacopoeia. Chinese ephedra (*Ephedra sinica*), used for asthma, and qinghao (*Artemisia*), used for malaria, are two such examples.

Innovations and publications during the Ming Dynasty broadened the scope of TCM. New theories in the etiology of disease and discoveries in anatomy appeared, as well as the formation of a system of treating communicable diseases which included the use of inoculation against smallpox—long before its use in Europe.

TCM continues to thrive in China. Hospitals and medical schools in China offer both Western and traditional Chinese medicine, and clinics typically have two pharmacies: one dispensing Western drugs, the other dispensing herbs. Patients can choose the sort of medicine they prefer. As in earlier centuries, the Chinese medical system encompasses a range of therapies, all based on the same fundamental concepts and principles; herbal medicine is only one--but the most common—of this range.

ANATOMY OF THE HUMAN BODY

Traditional Chinese medical theory sees the body as comprising 12 major channels through which the vital energy qi (氣, pronounced "hei" in Cantonese) flows and by blood vessels through which blood flows.

Qi and blood have different functions but are related. Vital energy is believed to be the "commander" of the blood: "Qi moves [then] blood flows". At the same time blood is the 'mother' of the vital energy by being its material basis.

The channels—the meridians of acupuncture (經)—and collaterals (絡) through which the qi flows connect the internal organs with superficial organs and tissues, and with each other. Thus the body is an organic whole. Of the 12 major channels, ten correspond to major internal organs and are considered to function in pairs. The solid, yin viscera are: heart, liver, spleen, lung and kidney; the hollow, yang bowels are: small intestine, gall bladder, stomach, large intestine, and urinary bladder. The remaining pair refer to the Pericardium (tissue surrounding the heart) and the Triple Burners, i.e., the three portions of the body cavity: above the waist; at the diaphragm and umbilicus; and below the umbilicus.

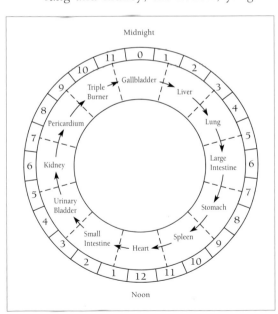

One interpretation of the flow of energy through the major channels (from The Essential Book of Traditional Chinese Medicine *by Liu Yanchi).*

3

P RINCIPLES OF CHINESE MEDICINE

CAUSES OF DISEASE

The fundamental root of all disease, according to traditional Chinese medicine, is an imbalance of yin and yang.

Yin (陰, pronounced "yum" in Cantonese) and yang (陽, "yeung" in Cantonese) is (not are) a philosophical concept referring to the fundamentally dichotomous nature of everything in the universe. Up/down, in/out, hot/cold, female/male—all are relative concepts which depend on contrast for definition. Any illness can be described in terms of an excess or deficiency in some dichotomy (yin/yang).

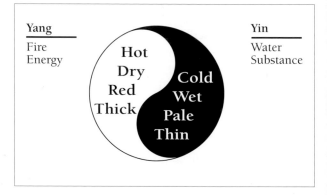

The two most common imbalances causing illness in the human body are, as with weather—heat/cold and wet/dry. Excess heat in the body is associated with redness and inflammation; skin infections, ulcers, and acne are examples. Cold in the body may manifest as poor digestion, poor circulation, diarrhea. Internal dampness causes diseases such as rheumatism and can give rise to wet, oozing skin conditions such as athlete's foot and eczema. Dryness, on the other hand, may manifest as dry skin, constipation, coughing.

Principles Of Treatment

"To treat a disease one should determine its root," directs the medical classic of the Yellow Emperor. There are two aspects of any disease: the fundamental, referring to the cause; and the incidental, referring to external symptoms. Which should be treated first depends on the severity of the symptoms and the patient's vital energy. Medical texts emphasize that symptoms change during the course of a disease and differ between patients. The same disease may have different symptoms, and different diseases may have the same symptoms. Hence, determining the fundamental cause is crucial to prescribing the correct remedy.

Once cause is determined, treatment can begin: "ming, bo, seh" (明、補、瀉): Understand [then] add [or] subtract. Particular therapies are chosen in order to replenish deficiencies (e.g., of heat or blood or vital energy) or to dissipate excesses.

The Role Of Herbs

Each herb (and food, for that matter) is considered to have a particular dynamic force (i.e., it may cause energy to ascend, descend, to move inward or outward), a particular flavor (sweet, sour, salty, bitter, or pungent), and an association with one or more of the energy channels and/or with qi or blood. Based on the diagnosis, herbs will be prescribed to bring about the desired effects.

I N Practice

Visiting The Doctor

In diagnosis, the traditional Chinese doctor follows a simple pattern of inspection (望診), listening (聞診), questioning (問診), and taking the patient's pulse (切診). No equipment is required except a small pillow on which the patient rests his arm during the pulse-taking.

Generally, in Hong Kong, doctors practice medicine in one of two ways: either in conjunction with a medicinal herb shop or independently. In the former case, the doctor will usually be seated at a desk at the back of the shop, with patients waiting in line.

When the doctor is independent, he may have a clinic or he may simply see patients in his home. Patients may be seen on a first come-first served basis; or by appointment; or, for the more famous doctors, by numbered ticket. A fixed number of tickets are given out in the morning; patients are then seen in the order of the numbered tickets.

Diagnosis typically begins with the patient's description of his complaint. As the person speaks, the doctor will be noting the general colour and condition of the skin; the manner of the patient (nervous, lethargic, depressed, etc.); any odours—that is, any clues as to how the body as a whole is functioning. Similarly the questions he asks will concern body function— bowel movements, digestion, perspiration, dietary habits. He will ask to see the tongue; its size, form, colour and coating all provide information.

Through this evidence the doctor will develop a picture of the patient's imbalances: which organs may be functioning in excess or may be deficient; the state of the blood and of vital energy, and hence what needs to be corrected to restore health. The doctor will then take the pulse to confirm or adjust his diagnosis.

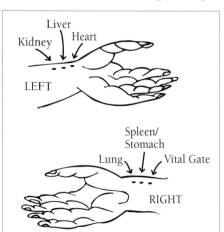

6

The pulse is taken at six positions on each of the wrists. Of these 12 positions, each corresponds to one of the internal organs and reflects by its nature the state of that organ. The doctor will seek to characterize the pulse in general, as well as individual organs. Entire treatises have been written on the qualities of the pulse; one of the classic texts describes 120 different forms. Twenty-eight kinds are commonly distinguished, with three predominant pairs of characteristics: floating or deep; slow or rapid; and weak or surging. Metaphor is used to describe particular types, e.g., taut like a violin string, irregular like chicken scratching, or slippery like beads rolling on a plate.

Having refined his diagnosis and determined the nature of the disease, the doctor will then write a prescription. Most prescriptions contain 5-20 ingredients, a combination custom-tailored for the patient's particular constitution and complex of symptoms. Each may be classified either as the principal, or as an adjuvant, auxiliary, or conductant ingredient. The principal ingredient provides the primary curative action; the adjuvant supports or strengthens the principal action; the auxiliary or correctant ingredient(s) relieve secondary symptoms or temper the action of the principal ingredient, and the conductant directs action to the affected channel or site. The doctor's prescription will include names and amounts of the herbs to be taken. The patient will be instructed how many times to take the prescription and when to return for the follow-up visit. For acute problems such as flu, a second visit is usually not necessary. For chronic conditions, many visits will be required, and the doctor will adjust the medicine to the patient's changing condition.

FILLING THE PRESCRIPTION

The next step for the patient is to have the prescription filled. Except when seeing doctors in medicinal herb shops, the patient is free to take his prescription anywhere.

In the shops, prescriptions are filled by weighing out the ingredients from the vast array of bottles and drawers of the various medicinal materials. The shopkeeper will spread large squares of paper on the counter—one sheet for each dose (one, two or three is common). He will then weigh the ingredients one by one, using hand-held scales, and dump them together on the papers. When done, he will recheck the list, fold up the papers, secure each with a rubber band, and pass them on to the cashier. Also included with each packet will be two preserved plums or rolls of dried hawthorn flakes ("saan zha bang"); these are to be taken as chasers after the medicine—which often turns out to be black and bitter. Using an abacus, the cost of the ingredients will be calculated, the total written on the prescription, and the bill presented to the patient. Subsequently, whenever the prescription is filled, the shop will tend to charge the price recorded on the prescription—even when it is filled at a different shop.

PREPARING THE MEDICINE

The next step is to prepare the medicine. This requires a special earthenware pot and 1-3 hours.

Pots used for boiling medicine are of a particular shape, and are always made of earthenware as metal can adversely affect some herbal constituents. Medicine pots can be identified by their small, uniform size (approximately 20 cm tall) and by the presence of both a handle and an angled spout attached to the body of the pot. The lids are flat, without holes. N.B. Soup pots have handles but no spouts and lids with a hole.

Ingredients of one packet are emptied into the pot; water is added. The doctor will have indicated the appropriate amount of water on the prescription, usually in numbers of rice bowls. For example, "Three bowls of water reduced to one" is a common directive.

The concoction is brought slowly to the boil, and then simmered until the liquid is reduced to the specified amount. The medicine is then poured out and, when cooled enough, drunk.

Each packet can be—and is usually—boiled twice in order to extract all its goodness. Many people boil up the herbs in the evening; pour out the liquid and take the first dose; leave the herbs in the pot; then next morning add water and boil them up again for the second dose. Alternatively, other people boil up the two doses one after the other, combine them then drink half in the evening and the other half the following morning. Or, for those too busy to boil medicine, for a small extra charge, the medicine shop will boil up the herbs. The customer tells the shop when he will be in, and the shop prepares the medicine, keeping it warm in a thermos until the customer arrives.

T HE MATERIA MEDICA

Traditional Chinese medicine shops typically stock 100-200 natural medicinal substances, commonly referred to as 'herbs', although they include minerals and items of animal origin. The selections depicted here represent some of the the most commonly and frequently used of these items.

FOODS AS MEDICINE

Among the herbs—both on these pages and in the shops themselves—are a number of items which seem to be food not medicine. Cantonese herb shops in Hong Kong, for example, often carry in conspicuous display such items as mushrooms (black mushrooms or shiitake, black ear fungus, white ear fungus), nuts (walnuts, cashews, peanuts), jujubes (red, brown and black), various dried beans, figs, barley, and abalone. Most of these items are key ingredients in the extensive soup cuisine of the Cantonese; others are simply exotic and expensive foodstuffs. The presence of foods in a medicine shop reflects, first, the Chinese belief that food and medicine are part of a continuous spectrum, varying in potency but not mode of action, and, secondly, the familiarity of ordinary people with these principles and their daily application.

PATENT MEDICINES

In addition to the loose herbs, Chinese herb shops also usually sell a wide range of patent medicines, both Western and Chinese. The Chinese patent medicines are, to use an analogy, like clothes bought off the rack rather than tailor-made. They are generally based on prescriptions which have been developed over decades, or even centuries, of use.

Descriptions on the boxes of what these medicines are used for can seem too broad to be true; this broadness is consistent with Chinese medical theory. A Chinese patent medicine will be devised to treat a symptom-complex such as "liver fire" or "damp wind"; each such complex will manifest in a variety of symptoms and in different ways according to the individual constitution. Hence, one looks for a combination of conditions, rather than an individual symptom, to choose a medicine.

TONIC TINCTURES

Another form of medicine occasionally on display in medicine shops are large (1-2 liter) jars full of herbs immersed in a dark liquid. These are special tonics, prepared by steeping complex combinations of herbs in rice wine for several months. There are three basic types: tonic for the yin essence ("bo yum"), tonic for the yang essence ("bo yeung"), and tonics for the elderly. Quite expensive, they are bought and drunk regularly, in small quantities.

THE COMMON HERBS

For easy reference, in the following descriptions:

* The herbs are divided into three **categories**—animal, plant, and mineral. Plant matter is further divided into three groups according to part of the plant used, i.e., underground stems and roots; flowers and leaves; and fruits, nuts, and seeds.
* Within each group, herbs are listed in **alphabetical order** according to the English name.
* Five **names** are given for each herb in this order: common English; botanical; Chinese characters; Pinyin Romanization of the Mandarin pronunciation, indicated by [**M**]; the Cantonese phonetic pronunciation, indicated by [**C**].
* **Action** refers to effect on the body. Generally this is described in terms of Chinese medical concepts. Reports from Western clinical research are preceded by [**CR**].
* **Use** refers to how the herbs are used—in, e.g., (medicinal) prescriptions, soups (to accompany meals), (sweet) dessert soups, or biscuits and confections.

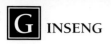 INSENG

GINSENG SPECIES

In ancient Chinese medical texts, ginseng was one of a group of medicinal herbs highly respected for their properties in regulating body function. We now know these properties to be due to chemical constituents similar to hormones. Today, three ginsengs are marketed, two of which belong to the genus Panax. "Panax" comes from the Greek "pan" meaning all and "akos" meaning to heal or to cure, hence a cure-all or panacea. Of the many species of this genus, native to both North America and Asia, the following three are most commonly cultivated and marketed:

Chinese or Korean ginseng (Panax ginseng)
高麗參 · 人參

[M] Gao li shen; [C] Go lai sum; yun sum
This is the most widely used and marketed of the Panax species, and is now cultivated in the northern parts of both China and Korea.

American ginseng (Panax quinquefolium)
花旗參

[M] Yang shen; [C] Fa kei sum
This grows wild on forested mountain slopes in eastern North America; the centre of cultivation is in Wisconsin.

Russian or Siberian ginseng (Eleutherococcus senticosus)
蘇聯 — 西伯利亞參（抽參）

[M] Chou shen ; [C] Chau sum
This herb belongs to another genus, albeit in the same family as true ginseng. Its chemistry and therapeutic properties are similar to true ginseng.

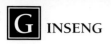

THERAPEUTIC PROPERTIES AND USES

In their respective native cultures, both Chinese and American ginsengs have been highly regarded and widely used as medicine. Interestingly, they have served in the treatment of many of the same ailments.

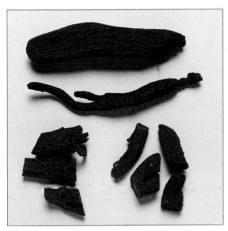

Chinese or Korean ginseng

In China, the use of ginseng has been recorded for more than 4000 years. Legend maintains that the fairies gave it to men; hence portrayals of fairies traditionally decorate boxes and advertisements, particularly for Korean products.

The uses of ginseng are almost as wide as its reputation. Chinese physicians have prescribed to treat medical conditions ranging from, e.g. dysentery, malaria, cancer, and diabetes, as well as to improve blood circulation; to reduce high blood pressure; and to remedy almost all blood and skin diseases, from pimples and boils to anemia. Known as the Herb of Eternal Life and the Elixir of Life among ordinary people, it is taken as a general tonic to lengthen and enhance life.

In sum, the fundamental value in ginseng is its extraordinary ability to detoxify and normalize the entire system—or, in the terms of Chinese medical theory, to increase vital energy. Like other "alteratives," it re-establishes the body's healthy functions, corrects disordered processes of nutrition and metabolism, and detoxifies or purifies the blood and lymphatic systems. It also works slowly and gently.

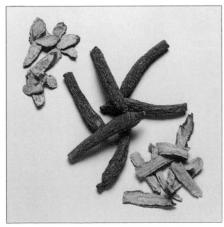

American ginseng

Research by Japanese, Chinese and Russian scientists since the mid-1900s has established the chemical basis for some of these remarkable properties. Many of ginseng's constituents are chemically unique, hence given names derived from the genus name. "Panacene" is one such constituent which is a tranquilizer and pain reliever; "panaxin" another, which stimulates the brain, improves muscle tone and tonifies the cardiovascular system. "Panquilon" stimulates the endocrine secretions (e.g., pituitary, thyroid and adrenal glands) which in turn regulate other body processes from digestion to aging. In addition, ginseng contains a range of B vitamins, significant amounts of minerals, and enzymes. Germanium is also a constituent which has been shown clinically effective in treating anemia (by stimulating the formation of red blood cells in bone marrow) and is being investigated as a cure for cancer.

In Hong Kong, Korean and American ginseng are used specifically and quite differently. American ginseng is considered to be best for general purposes--for both acute and chronic conditions--because it is more generally nourishing and has fewer side effects. Korean ginseng, on the other hand, is used in cases of "yang deficiency". Hence, old men (yang diminishes naturally with age) during winter (a very yin season) particularly find it beneficial. If yang is over-stimulated—e.g., if taken by young people or in summer—"hot" symptoms such as headache, mouth ulcers and insomnia can result.

PROCESSING AND MARKETING

Ginseng root is sold in an assortment of forms, from whole roots to processed medicines, candies and even cosmetics. American ginseng is generally sold as short lengths of the dried root or as fine slices.

Processing of Korean ginseng (whether from China or from Korea) is more complicated, and depends on the origin (wild or cultivated), age, method and place of production. In all cases the first step is the same: fresh roots are carefully dug and gently brushed to remove soil without damaging the delicate rootlets.

WHITE ginseng refers to roots less than six years old. Considered second quality, they are bleached with sulfur gas and sun-dried—and seldom exported from Korea.

RED ginseng must be at least four, but is usually more than six, years old. The various methods of processing generally involve steam-heating for several hours and a final drying over low heat or in the sun. The finest whole roots are bound with fine white string—to keep all the rootlets intact.

Tips On Purchase

For both American and Korean ginseng, the untouched, whole root or root pieces are the best buy. Having the skin intact is critical to quality because ginseng's most valuable constituents lie in the dark, exterior skin. The larger and the more the Korean roots resemble a human form the more costly they are. Nevertheless, the far cheaper rootlets ("sum so" in Cantonese) may—actually, chemically--be more powerful because the surface-to-volume ratio is larger and they are unlikely to have been scraped.

Tips On Use

When taking ginseng, avoid taking Vitamin C (including fresh fruits), avoid eating cooked radish, and never drink tea at the same time. All three will reduce the efficacy of the ginseng. Furthermore, it is not recommended to take Korean ginseng every day to avoid "overheating" the body. American ginseng is more appropriate as a daily tonic over an extended period. (See recipe for American ginseng tea, p.50, and Korean ginseng soup, p.48.)

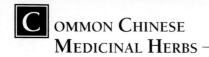

**R
O
O
T
S**

**A
N
D**

**S
T
E
M
S**

Achyranthes (*Achyranthes bidentata*) 牛膝
[M] Niu xi; [C] Ngau chut

Action: Redistributes fire energy (heat) downward.

Use: Prescriptions; congee, soups.

Remarks: Like rhubarb, this herb directs energy downward. Where rhubarb primarily affects the digestive system, achyranthes primarily affects blood circulation—particularly to the lower extremities. Hence it is used in winter tonics when symptoms include cold feet. N.B. Both this and rhubarb are contraindicated for pregnant women, as the downward moving energy can induce abortion.

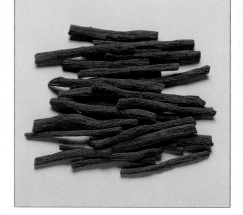

Angelica (*Angelica sinensis*) 當歸
[M] Dang quai; [C] Dong gwai

Action: Nourishes the blood and yin; moisturizes the large intestine; regulates menstruation. [CR] Contains vitamin B12 and aids blood formation.

Use: Prescriptions; patent drugs; soups.

Remarks: This is considered the queen of women's herbs, able to tonify and invigorate the entire female system. It is also used in treating blood deficiency, diabetes, and rheumatic pains, in both men and women.

Angelica has a distinctive penetrating fragrance, reminiscent of celery (both are in the same botanical

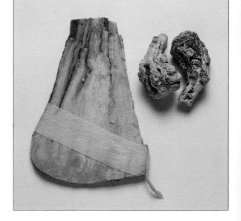

family). This smell is one measure of its quality. As illustrated it is sold in two forms: as slices of large roots which are primarily used for prescriptions; and as small whole nobs which are preferred for making soup.

Baizhu *(Atractylodes macrocephala)* 白朮

[M] Bai zhu; [C] Baak soot

Action: Revitalizes the spleen; aids urination and reduces perspiration, particularly night sweats; protects the liver; sedates fetus in threatened abortion. [CR] Increases secretion of bile and gastric juices; promotes adrenal cortex function.

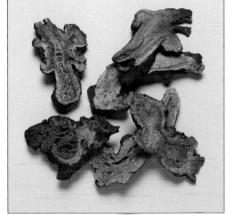

Use: Soups, particularly in summer and particularly in combination with China-root.

Remarks: This is a gentle herb, used— in small doses—even for babies and small children. The best are those from Yu-chien in Chekiang province.

China-Root *(Poria cocos)* 茯苓

[M] Fu ling; [C] Fook ling

Action: Facilitates movement of fluids (blood, lymph, etc.), hence used particularly for kidney and bladder problems. Also improves spleen function, regulates the stomach, tranquilizes the nerves. [CR] Diuretic.

Use: Prescriptions; soups; biscuits.

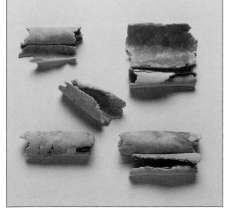

Remarks: This is the fruiting body of a mushroom which grows underground— like truffles—on the roots of certain pine trees. It occurs worldwide, particularly in Yunnan province (which is reputed to produce the best for medicinal purposes) and in eastern North America where it is variously known as tuckahoe, Indian bread or Virginia truffle. It is sweet and bland in taste and mild in nature. Smaller younger ones, particularly those with a bit of the host root attached, are considered superior and are called [M] fu shen or [C] fook sun (伏神).

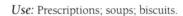

R
O
O
T
S

A
N
D

S
T
E
M
S

17

Chinese Cornbind (*Polygonum multiflorum*) 首烏

[M] Shou wu; [C] Sau wu

Action: Nourishes the blood and kidneys; moisturizes the large intestine.

Use: Prescriptions, alone or in combinations; desserts.

Remarks: Both men and women use this herb frequently, particularly as they grow older. By nourishing the cardiovascular system it helps reduce high blood pressure and hardening of the arteries. By nourishing the kidneys it slows the greying of hair.

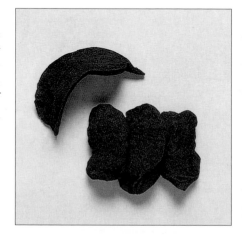

Chinese Foxglove

(*Rehmannia glutinosa*) 地黃

[M] Di huang; [C] Dei wong

Action: Nourishes the yin. In addition, the raw form (生地, [C] Sang dei) cools the blood, while the cooked form (熟地, [C] Sook dei) tonifies the blood.

Use: Prescriptions; soups.

Remarks: This is a common ingredient in women's prescriptions. Both raw and cooked forms are black, mashed preparations of the root of the plant. Cooking involves repeated steaming and drying of the root mixed with other ingredients including yellow rice or millet wine, Chinese cardamom, and tangerine peel.

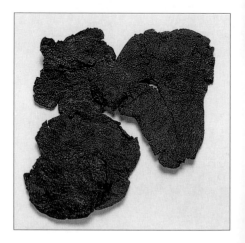

Chinese Yam (*Dioscorea opposita*) 山藥・淮山

[M] Shan yao; [C] Wai saan

Action: Invigorates the yang, especially of the kidneys, hence increases production of semen; tonic to the spleen and stomach. [CR] Related species contain steroid and progesterone precursors; can lower blood cholesterol and blood pressure.

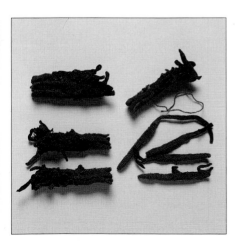

Use: Prescriptions; soups; biscuits.

Remarks: As a tonic to the digestive system, this is a common and quite palatable ingredient in soups, used year round, particularly paired with wolfberries (q.v.). In its capacity to regulate the body's sugar level, it is used in diabetes. Less well known is its role as a tonic to the male reproductive system. Ancient texts describe Chinese yam as the all-around yang counterpart to angelica (q.v.).

Cordyceps (*Cordyceps sinensis*)
冬蟲夏草

[M] Dong chong xia cao; [C] Doeng choeng ha cho

Action: Nourishes the yang of the kidneys; invigorates the yin of the lungs.

Use: Prescriptions; soups; desserts.

Remarks: This unusual—and expensive —herb is highly valued for its unusual ability to nourish both yin and yang. Hence it is particularly recommended in convalescence, for growing children, and for the elderly.

Its origin is equally remarkable. The herb is a fungus that consumes the larvae of a particular bat moth as the larvae overwinters in the soil (of Sichuan and Tibet). Hence, what begins in winter (dong) as a worm (chong) by summer (xia/ha) is vegetable matter (cao/cho).

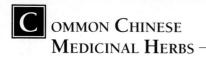

Dangshen (*Codonopsis* spp.) 黨參

[M] Dang shen; [C] Dong sum

Action: Tonifies vital energy, particularly acting on the spleen which in turn regulates metabolism; toughens muscles and bones.

Use: Prescriptions; soups.

Remarks: Ancient medical texts include this as one of the seven "shen" which, like ginseng, have hormone-like properties in being able to regulate physiological processes. Grown in several provinces, the best is from Fanghsien in Hupeh, known commonly in Cantonese as "fong dong". It is used year-round (see recipe for the soup "Ng Gwun Tong", p.49).

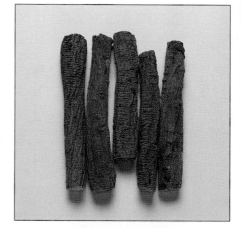

Eucommia (*Eucommia ulmoides*) 杜仲

[M] Du zhong; [C] Do joeng

Action: Nourishes the yang, especially of the kidneys, hence strengthening the waist and loin region; calms the embryo during pregnancy. [CR] Reduces absorption of cholesterol and alleviates atheriosclerosis; can lower blood pressure.

Use: Prescriptions; soups; patent medicines; poultices.

Remarks: This is a potent herb, particularly used externally to treat sprains and bruises (i.e., ruptured tissues) and to alleviate symptoms of kidney deficiency, e.g., lumbago,

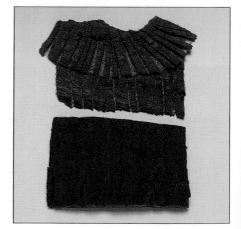

dizziness, impotence and fatigue. Before use, the bark is scored in deep parallel lines, exposing white strands of latex. In the illustration, an entire piece is shown below and a cut piece, above.

Ginger (dried) *(Zingiber officinale)* 乾薑

[M] Gon jiang; [C] Gon geung

Action: Warms the lungs, promotes circulation, pushes wind down and out of the digestive system. [CR] Alleviates nausea in post-operative patients; any form of ginger seems effective.

Use: Prescriptions.

Remarks: Fresh and dried ginger are considered to have similar effects, differing only in strength. The milder, fresh form (left) is used widely in small quantities in general cooking and in larger quantities in preparing remedies for colds and nausea. The dried form (right) is used in prescriptions for more severe problems of coldness in the internal regions.

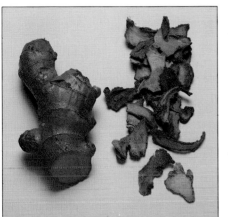

Golden Thread *(Coptis chinensis)* 黃蓮

[M] Huang lian; [C] Wong leen

Action: Detoxifies; clears heat from all major internal organs, especially the large intestines and heart. [CR] Promotes bile secretion; has broad-spectrum action against bacteria and protozoa.

Use: Prescriptions; infusions for washing infections and sore eyes; patent medicines.

Remarks: This is a potent, bitter herb commonly and primarily used in cases of dysentery and food poisoning, particularly when accompanied by symptoms of 'heat' such as headache and red face.

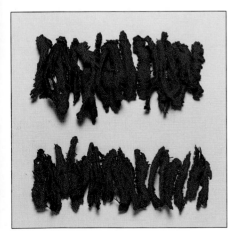

ROOTS AND STEMS

Licorice *(Glycyrrhiza uralensis)* 甘草
[M] Gan cao; [C] Gum cho

Action: Its energy enters all meridians, benefits all organs; like a buffer, it can enhance the beneficial action and reduce the toxicity of other herbs. [CR] Raises blood pressure; has estrogen-like constituents and properties.

Use: Prescriptions; used in the preparation of preserved fruits.

Remarks: This is arguably the most commonly used herb in China. Because of its unique property of affecting all 12 major meridians, one or two slices appear in many prescriptions. It is virtually universally used in preparing preserved fruits.

In Europe a different species (*Glycyrrhiza glabra*) occurs which is similarly used in medicine (particularly as a uterine tonic and for bronchial complaints) as well as in preparing licorice candy.

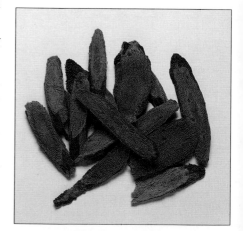

Lily Bulbs *(Lilium lancifolium)* 百合
[M] Bai he; [C] Baat hup

Action: Clears lung fire; nourishes yin.

Use: Prescriptions; soups, both sweet and savory.

Remarks: Valued as one of the few herbs which can nourish the yin of the kidneys, this is nonetheless so mild as to be more of a food than a medicine. It is

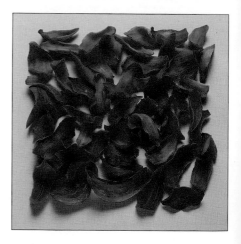

common in soups year round, from the general tonic "Ching Bo Leung" (see recipe, p.47) to sweet soups, particularly those with red beans. (N.B. Fresh bulbs are also sold, and are eaten raw or lightly cooked).

Milk Vetch (*Astragalus* spp.) 黃芪 · 北芪

[M] Huang qi; [C] Wong kei; but kei

Action: Invigorates and builds vital energy. [CR] Increases the number of white blood cells and regulates blood pressure.

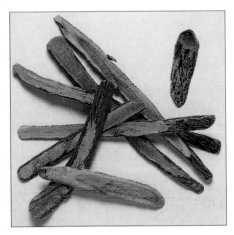

Use: Medicines; in soups, particularly as a pair with dangshen (q.v.).

Remarks: This is a favorite tonic for fatigue due to stress and for nervous exhaustion evidenced by emotional instability. The central portion of the root is yellow (hence the Cantonese name "wong"), and it comes from the northern provinces (hence the name "but"). Larger roots are considered more effective.

Notoginseng (*Panax notoginseng*) 三七 · 田七

[M] San qi; [C] Saam chut; teen chut

Action: Internally, promotes circulation and dissolves clots; an effective analgesic. Externally, haemostatic when applied to wounds.

Use: Prescriptions; soups; patent medicines.

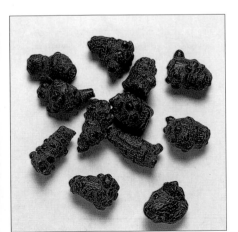

Remarks: This is an important herb for treating traumatic injuries because of its ability to stop bleeding. The highly regarded "Yunnan Bai Yao", of which notoginseng is the main ingredient, has been used for centuries, particularly by soldiers. Both this and the various true ginsengs are different species of the same genus. When used in soups, this has health-restoring properties similar to ginseng.

R
O
O
T
S

A
N
D

S
T
E
M
S

Peony (*Paeonia moutan*) 牡丹皮

[M] Mu dan pi; [C] Mao daan pei

Action: Clears blood heat and restores proper circulation. [CR] Lowers blood pressure; has broad-spectrum anti-bacterial activity and anti-inflammatory activity.

Use: Prescriptions.

Remarks: This herb is highly respected and widely used for any problem relating to blood, from menstrual difficulties to problems of circulation. It is also particularly potent for relieving sinus allergy problems.

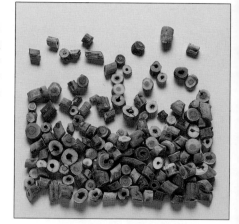

Rhubarb (*Rheum officinale*) 大黃

[M] Da huang; [C] Dai wong

Action: Purgative; detoxifies the digestive system, clears heat from the entire body, pushing it down and out through the digestive system, hence a laxative or purgative depending on the dose.

Use: Prescriptions; patent medicines.

Remarks: While rhubarb leaf stalks are a vegetable in the West, only the root is used in China. In adults, it is used for constipation and jaundice; in children it is used to eliminate worms.

N.B. Rhubarb is contraindicated for pregnant women, as the downward moving energy can induce abortion.

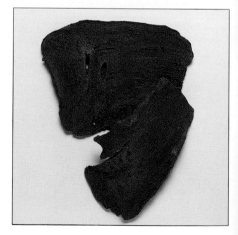

Solomon's Seal (*Polygonatum odoratum*) 玉竹

[M] Yu zhu; [C] Yook jook

Action: Nourishes the yin of the lungs and stomach; good for dry cough and loss of appetite due to over-worked stomach. [CR] Promotes heart function; excess lowers blood pressure.

Use: Prescriptions; soups; patent medicines.

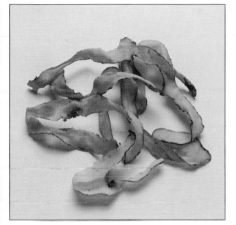

Remarks: This is a common soup ingredient, almost invariably associated with heat and dryness—either in the weather or in the body. With mild flavor and effects, it is appropriate for family use year-round.

White Mulberry (branches)

(*Morus alba*) 桑枝

[M] Sang zhi; [C] Song jee

Action: Redistributes vital energy in the upper part of the body.

Use: Prescriptions; congee.

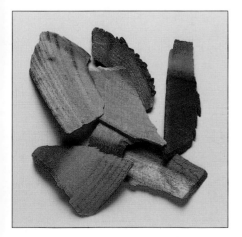

Remarks: This herb is considered a "conductant", or distributor, for the upper body. This means it can bring energy of other herbs to the torso and, particularly, to the arms when needed in that region. Hence it is commonly included in prescriptions for rheumatism and when symptoms include cold hands.

L
E
A
V
E
S

A
N
D

F
L
O
W
E
R
S

Chrysanthemum (flowers) (*Chrysanthemum morifolium*) 菊花
[M] Ju hua; [C] Gook fa

Action: Generally eliminates heat from the body and detoxifies; with anti-bacterial and anti-viral action. [CR] Lowers blood pressure and cholesterol when used alone as a tea.

Use: Prescriptions; tea.

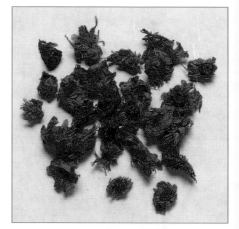

Remarks: Chrysanthemum is widely consumed in summer because it can cool and detoxify the internal organs (particularly the liver) without adversely affecting the stomach. Cantonese restaurants serve red tea ([M] pu erh; [C] bo lei) infused with chrysanthemum flowers making the beverage known as "gook bo", which is considered a balanced yin-yang combination. Another common combination is chrysanthemum and honeysuckle, which is both drunk and used as a wash for minor skin infections and abscesses.

Corn Silk (*Zea mays*) 玉米鬚
[M] Yu mi xu; [C] Sook mai so

Action: Invigorates vital energy of pancreas and kidney. [CR] Lowers blood sugar; increases secretion of bile; clears gallbladder of stones; relieves edema; lowers blood pressure.

Use: Prescriptions; soups.

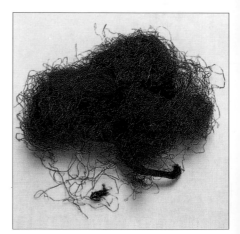

Remarks: Useful for diabetics, this is also considered effective in eliminating stones in the kidney and gall bladder when used consistently in an extended course of treatment.

Dandelion *(Taraxacum officinale)* 蒲公英

[M] Pu gong ying; [C] Po gong ying

Action: Clears blockages in energy paths in the body, especially those associated with the liver and stomach; reduces inflammation. [CR] The root has been shown to stimulate bile secretion (hence useful in cases of hepatitis, gallstones) and urea excretion.

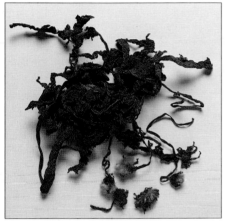

Use: Prescriptions.

Remarks: Although the Chinese use the leaves while Western herbalists use the root, all parts of the dandelion appear to have similar constituents and effects. Its characteristically bitter principles cleanse, stimulate and tonify all of the glands involved with digestion and particularly the liver. Hence, Chinese doctors generally prescribe dandelion to counteract poison as represented by, e.g., boils, skin abscesses, chest congestion, or cancer.

Downy Artemesia

(Artemisia capillaris) 茵陳

[M] Yin chuen; [C] Yan chun

Action: Facilitates urination, i.e., helps eliminate wet heat; regulates liver function, hence useful for jaundice of all causes. [CR] Promotes bile secretion.

Use: Prescriptions.

Remarks: In earlier eras, traditional families fed a sweet tea made from this and honeysuckle to children once a week to prevent jaundice. It is still commonly used to treat jaundice and a range of other liver problems.

**L
E
A
V
E
S

A
N
D

F
L
O
W
E
R
S**

Ephedra (Ephedra sinensis) 麻黃
[M] Ma huang; [C] Ma wong

Action: Associated with lungs and urinary bladder, it opens pores to expel external evils trapped inside. [CR] Contains ephedrine which acts like adrenaline but with more long-lasting effects.

Use: Prescriptions; patent drugs.

Remarks: The most important use of this herb is in treating asthmatic attacks. It is also used to induce sweating to eliminate fever of colds, and to facilitate complete eruption of measles. As it is appropriate for use only in cold weather, it is used more commonly in northern than southern China.

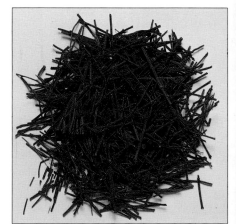

Honeysuckle (flowers)
(Lonicera japonica) 金銀花
[M] Jin yin hua; [C] Gum ngun fa

Action: Generally detoxifies and clears heat from the body. [CR] Has broad-spectrum antibiotic properties.

Use: Prescriptions; patent drugs; singly, as a tea; recently, as an injection.

Remarks: This is most commonly used together with forsythia, and this pair is the basis of a popular anti-flu pill.

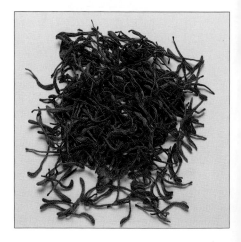

Loquat (leaves) *(Eriobotrya japonica)* 枇杷葉

[M] Pi pa yeh; [C] Pei pa yeep

Action: Particularly associated with the lungs, used to clear lung heat and eliminate phlegm, hence as an expectorant. [CR] Both leaves and fruits have been shown to

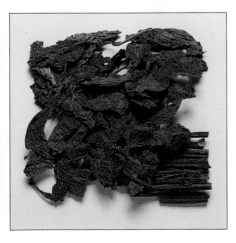

inhibit growth of the bacteria *Staphylococcus aureus* (cause of serious bronchial infections) and of flu virus.

Use: Prescriptions; patent cough syrups.

Remarks: This is the basis of one of the most popular and respected cough syrups available. Called "pei pa go", it is a combination of herbs in a base of honey and is taken by the spoonful to soothe irritated respiratory membranes.

Mint *(Mentha arvensis)* 薄荷

[M] Bo he; [C] Bok haw

Action: Clears heat and wind, eliminates phlegm, stops vomiting; alleviates itching which accompanies rashes, particularly when due to "wind-heat." [CR] Mint's essential oils have been shown to normalize digestive contractions, and to inhibit the growth of many important pathogenic micro-organisms, including influenza viruses, herpes, *Staphylococcus*, and candida.

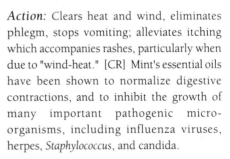

Use: Prescriptions.

Remarks: Mint has been used by folk cultures around the world--North and South America, Europe, Asia, Africa, Australia. It is best known as a stomach remedy for both chronic and acute problems. While it is a culinary herb in some cultures, the Chinese use it dried as a medicine, and only rarely fresh in cooking.

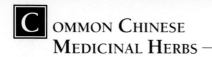

L
E
A
V
E
S

A
N
D

F
L
O
W
E
R
S

Self-Heal *(Prunella vulgaris)* 夏枯草

[M] Xia ku cao; [C] Ha gu cho

Action: Clears heat from the liver, thereby reducing heat and toxins in the blood.

Use: Prescriptions; singly, as a tea; soups.

Remarks: This is considered to be an excellent general tonic during the summer when heat-stress of the liver can generate a range of symptoms, such as headache, dizziness, and sore eyes.

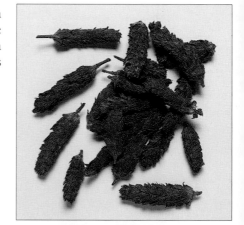

Tree Cotton *(flowers)*

(Bombax ceiba) 木棉花

[M] Mu mien hua; [C] Mook meen fa

Action: Diuretic; clears excessive heat from internal organs.

Use: Soups; drinks.

Remarks: These large red flowers are used almost exclusively in Southern China, where the tree is abundant in the wild. They are an essential ingredient in the "chasing dampness" soup combination, "Hui Sup Liu" (see recipe, p.48), as well as in Five Flower Tea. Both of these are taken in the summer to help regulate kidney function during hot, humid weather.

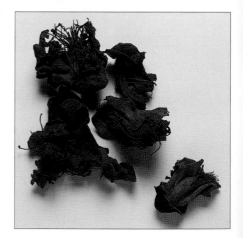

Adzuki Beans *(Phaseolus calcaratus)* 赤小豆

[M] Chi xiao dou; [C] Chek siu dau

Action: Diuretic; dispersing swellings by detoxifying.

Use: Soups.

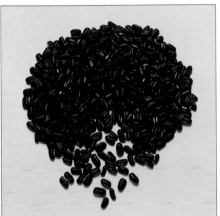

Remarks: This bean is highly regarded among the Cantonese and is common in household use for its ability to regulate water within the body, particularly expelling excess. Previously it was also prescribed for women's problems during and after pregnancy.

N.B. This is not the red bean ([C] "hoeng dau") used for sweet soups and fillings of pastries.

Apricot Kernels *(Prunus armeniaca)* 杏仁

[M] Xing ren; bitter, ku xing ren; [C] Hung yun.

Action: Moisturizes the lungs and large intestines; relieves spasmodic coughing. [CR] Contains laetrile, a controversial anti-carcinogenic compound.

Use: Prescriptions; soups, both sweet and savory.

Remarks: The Cantonese "naam but hung" is a mixture of the large sweet southern ("naam") kernels and the small bitter northern ("but") kernels. It is widely used in savory soups (e.g., with pork, carrots, radishes and figs) and in sweet dessert soups (particularly ground to a paste with rice flour), and is consumed particularly during the dry autumn and winter to lubricate the respiratory membranes.

Dates (*Zizyphus jujuba*) 棗

Black Dates: [M] Nan zao; [C] Naam jo 南棗
Red Dates: [M] Hong zao; [C] Hoeng jo 紅棗
Brown or Honey Dates: [M] Mi zao; [C] Mut jo 蜜棗

Action: Black dates tonify the yang of the stomach and spleen; red dates tonify the yang of the circulatory system; brown dates, sweetened with honey, moisten the internal organs.

Use: Prescriptions; soups; teas; confections.

Remarks: All three dates come from one species of shrub; differences in colour, flavour and medicinal value derive from processing and variety characteristics. The black date (upper right) is the most medicinal of the three. It is included in prescriptions, and almost invariably accompanies angelica, complementing

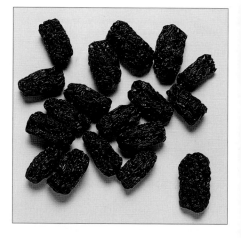

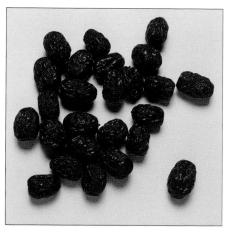

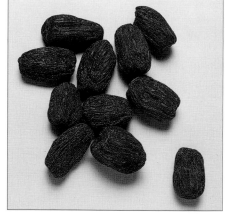

and enhancing that herb's action. The red date (left) is used in savory soups and braised dishes; further north in China it is eaten as a snack. The brown date (bottom right)—least medicinal of the three—is added to winter soups for sweetness and moisturizing effects, and is also used in candies and sweetmeats.

Cannabis (roasted seeds) *(Cannabis sativa)* 火麻仁

[M] Huo ma ren; [C] Foh ma yun

Action: Stimulates intestinal secretion of mucus and peristalsis; reduces water absorption; nourishes the yin and the spleen qi. Laxative in large doses; poisonous in overdoses.

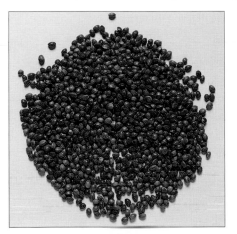

Use: Prescriptions; patent medicines; drinks.

Remarks: All parts of the hemp plant have been used in Chinese medicine for thousands of years. This herb is the roasted seeds; they may be eaten as they are but, more commonly are either boiled in prescriptions or ground, filtered and boiled to make a sweet, white drink commonly sold by herbal tea and dessert shops by the cup. In all preparations, this herb is used to moisturize the internal organs, particularly the intestines (hence relieving constipation).

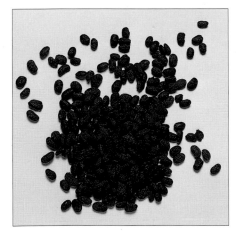

Fermented Black Soy Beans

(Glycine max: preparation) 淡豆豉

[M] Dan dou chi; [C] Taam dau see

Action: Induces perspiration thereby eliminating heat trapped in the interior of the body (particularly the lungs).

Use: Prescriptions.

Remarks: These are not the "fermented black soy beans" commonly used in cooking. Although, like their culinary counterpart, these are fermented the process differs, particularly in not involving salt.

Figs *(Ficus carica)* 無花果

[M] Wu hua guo; [C] Mo fa gwoh

Action: Moistens the lungs and the colon.

Use: Soups; desserts.

Remarks: The Cantonese add figs to savory soups and sweet dessert soups for flavour, aroma, and the fruit's ability to moisturize the lungs and the large intestines. Hence, it can stop coughing due to dryness and alleviate constipation.

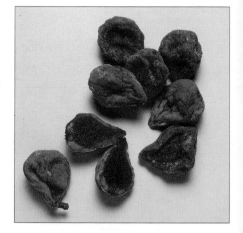

Forsythia *(Forsythia suspensa)* 連翹

[M] Lian qiao; [C] Leen kiu

Action: Clears heat, detoxifies. [CR] Component forsythol has broad spectrum anti-bacterial effects; contains bioflavonoids (also known previously as vitamin P) which helps skin pores to fight infection.

Use: Prescriptions; patent medicines.

Remarks: This is most famously, commonly, and effectively used in combination with honeysuckle flowers —the combination being known as "ngun kiu"—to relieve heat in the early stages of flu.

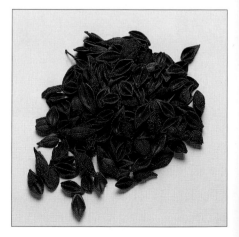

Foxnut *(Euryale ferox)* 茨實

[M] Qian shi; [C] Chee sut

Action: Invigorates the vital energy of the kidney.

Use: Soups.

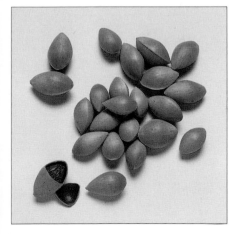

Remarks: Common, this is considered comparable to lotus nuts, which are in fact its close botanical relatives. They are mild in flavour, used year-round in meat and fish soups as well as the tonic "Ching Bo Leung" (see recipe, p.47).

Ginkgo Nuts *(Ginkgo biloba)* 白果

[M] Bai guo; [C] Baak gwoh

Action: Clears lung heat, reduces secretion of liquids in renal and reproductive systems.

Use: Desserts; congee; soups.

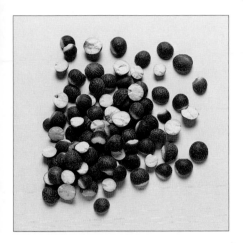

Remarks: This is the seed of one of the most ancient plants in the world--found only in cultivation. The raw seed is extremely toxic; the cure for poisoning is the shell of the seed.

Ginkgo extract now being sold for stimulating mental activity is prepared from the leaves, not the seeds.

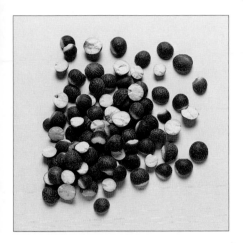

F
R
U
I
T
S
,
N
U
T
S
A
N
D
S
E
E
D
S

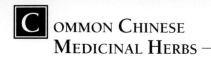

Hawthorn *(Crataegus pinnatifida)* 山楂
[M] Shan zha; [C] Saan ja

Action: Improves appetite and digestion by moving stagnant excess food. [CR] Lowers serum cholesterol and blood pressure; especially beneficial in cases of coronary artery blockage.

Use: Prescriptions; soups; snacks.

Remarks: Whole dried fruits are used in medicine and drinks, particularly paired with dried wheat or barley sprouts, [C] "mut nga". Macerated fruits are also made into wafers eaten as a snack--or as the sweet chaser eaten after a bitter bowl of medicine.

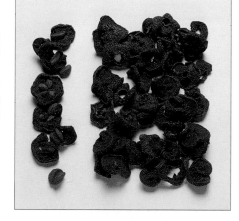

Hyacinth Beans *(Dolichos lablab)*
扁豆

[M] Bian dou; [C] Been dau

Action: Strengthens the vital energy of the spleen, hence enhancing the flow of body fluids.

Use: Soups.

Remarks: Also and perhaps more commonly known as lablab bean, a native of India, this is an item which the Cantonese use exclusively but commonly in summer soups. It can help the body regain energy and maintain fluid balance when perspiring heavily, as during hot humid weather. Actually, it is the skin of the bean which is the most powerful medicinally, and this can be bought separately as [C] "been dau yee".

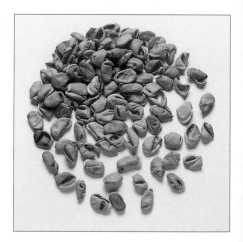

Job's Tears Barley *(Coix lachryma-jobi)* 苡米仁 · 薏米
[M] Yi yi ren; [C] Yee mai

Action: Diuretic, decongestant, detoxifying, anti-dysenteric.

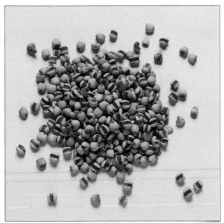

Use: Soups, savory and sweet.

Remarks: This is a humble but powerful herb used in a wide range of Cantonese soups for its general ability to help the body detoxify. It is particularly prescribed for boils and acne, for edema, and for tumors in the abdominal region.

Lingzhi *(Lucida ganoderma)* 靈芝
[M] Ling zhi; [C] Ling jee

Action: A general tonifier which regulates the qi of all the internal organs; enhances the immune system by increasing the power of T cells and macrophages; regulates cholesterol.

Use: Teas; patent medicines.

Remarks: This is one of the widely revered and commonly used health-restoring herbs. The name has ancient and auspicious connotations, as "zhi" (芝) is defined in the classics as the plant of immortality. Today the herb is primarily thought of in the treatment or tonification of the liver. It can be used daily, except by those suffering from "exopathic" conditions such as flu and fever or from excess fire due to yin deficiency.

Longan Fruit (*Euphoria longan*) 圓肉

[M]Yun rou; [C] Yoon yoek

Action: Nourishes and increases the production of blood; invigorates spleen qi.

Use: Prescriptions; soups; desserts; confections; drinks.

Remarks: This is highly recommended for insomnia. In the autumn and winter, a little is added to different teas and soups (e.g., American ginseng tea, Ng Gwun Tong, and Ching Bo Leung--see recipes) to nourish the fire in the "triple warmer".

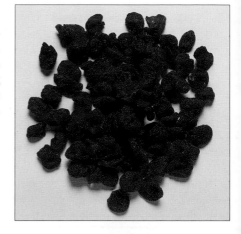

Lotus Seed Pods (*Nelumbo nucifera*) 蓮房

[M] Lian fung; [C] Leen fung

Action: Cleanses and enhances the functions of the urinary/reproductive systems; removes internal blood clots; can also be used externally to stop bleeding.

Use: Prescriptions; soups; patent medicines.

Remarks: This is particularly powerful in cleansing the urinary and reproductive systems in both men and women. It is used to stop profuse bleeding in menstruation. More recently it is being used in treating cervical cancer. Charcoal made from the pods is effective in healing herpes infections.

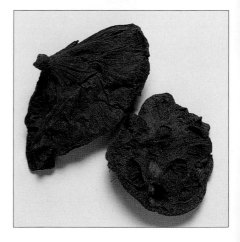

Lotus Seeds *(Nelumbo nucifera)* 蓮子

[M] Lian zi; [C] Leen jee

Action: Invigorates the vital energy of the kidney; balances heart-fire and kidney-water.

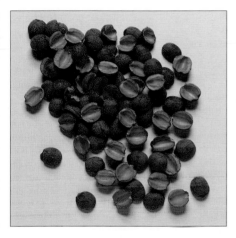

Use: Soups; desserts; rice dishes.

Remarks: Lotus seeds are associated with festivals, and most commonly used in sweets—sweet soups, rice desserts (i.e., Eight Treasure Rice), and snacks. Cooked and mashed, lotus seed paste is a traditional filling for mooncakes and other pastries.

Mandarin Tangerine Peel

(Citrus reticulata) 陳皮

[M] Chen pi; [C] Chun pei

Action: Invigorates the qi of the spleen, which in turn regulates fluids in the body, eliminating excess dampness and phlegm.

Use: Prescriptions; soups (sweet and savory); meat and vegetable dishes; preserved fruits.

Remarks: The best quality are light in weight, dark in colour, and old. They impart rich, mellow flavour and fragrance and are believed to enhance digestibility of foods with which they are cooked. During tangerine season, the peels of this particular species cost far more than the fruit, as many housewives dry their own, keeping them for years until properly aged.

F
R
U
I
T
S
,
N
U
T
S
A
N
D
S
E
E
D
S

Peach Kernels (Prunus persica) 桃仁

[M] Tao ren; [C] To yun

Action: Invigorates the yang of the kidneys and clears blockages in the energy channels, restoring energy and fluid movement throughout the body, hence a mild laxative and diuretic.

Use: Prescriptions; dessert soups.

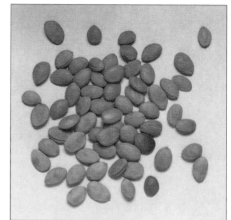

Remarks: This herb falls in the category of those able to "manage and discipline the blood." Hence it is used to treat forms of amenorrhea and dysmenorrhea which arise from blockage in circulation, certain traumatic injuries, and some cases of high blood pressure. Similarly, it is not prescribed for pregnant women because the fetus represents a blockage of the mother's energy flow and could be lost as the channels are cleared.

Pearl Barley (Hordeum vulgare) 大麥 · 洋苡米

[M] Da mai; [C] Yeung yee mai

Action: Invigorates spleen yang; decongestant, refrigerant, diuretic.

Use: Soups; desserts.

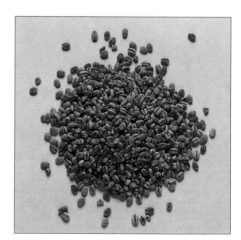

Remarks: Like Job's tears barley, pearl barley is most commonly used in soups during hot humid weather for its ability to cool and dry out the body. It can stop muscular spasms due to dampness trapped in the body.

Wheat *(Triticum aestivum)* 小麥

[M] Xiao mai; [C] Siu mut

Action: Sedative; calms the heart; stops sweating.

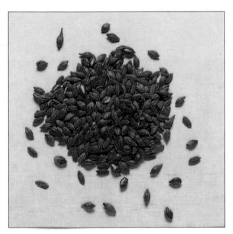

Use: Prescriptions; desserts; drinks.

Remarks: Rich in B vitamins, this is used to moderate nervous energy, e.g. to control hyperactivity, to alleviate constant anxiety, to calm hysteria (particularly in women). The whole mature kernels are used; those which float in water are reputed to be the most effective.

Wolfberry *(Lycium chinense)* 枸杞子

[M] Ji zi; [C] Gau gei jee

Action: Nourishes the liver yin and, therefore, also the eyes; improves function of spleen (hence blood formation) and kidneys (associated with bones and virility).

Use: Prescriptions; soups (savory and sweet); singly, as tea.

Remarks: An important traditional tonic, this is very common in soups, both savory and sweet, often paired with dried Chinese yam ([C] "wai saan"). While generally used by women, an old Chinese saying warns men, "Do not take wolfberry when far away from home," ostensibly referring to the herb's ability to arouse sexual desire.

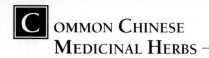
A
N
I
M
A
L

M
A
T
T
E
R

Abalone (Haliotis spp.) 鮑魚

[M] Bao yu; [C] Bao yu

Action: Nourishes the kidneys and liver yin.

Use: Soups.

Remarks: Abalone is a food whose gastronomic status as a delicacy overshadows—or perhaps enhances— its value as a medicinal tonic. The meat is an effective tonic; however, it is the shell which is the more traditional medicine. Abalone shell is prescribed for cataracts due to its ability to soften mineral accretions, and for cirrhosis of the liver.

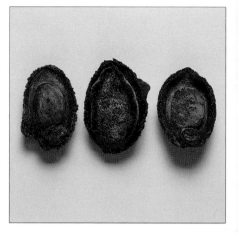

Bird's Nest (Collocalia sp.: preparation) 燕窩

[M] Yen wo; [C] Yeen woh

Action: Effective in convalescence, aids digestion and absorption; slows aging.

Use: Soups, savory and sweet; desserts.

Remarks: The commercial article is indeed a nest—"built" by certain sea swallows, native to Southeast Asia. Rather than collecting twigs and debris, these birds secrete a gelatinous substance from a gland in their mouths. This substance hardens into the matrix of the nest and is used to affix the nest to the ceilings and walls of the caves where they live. (As with superglue, the birds can get stuck to the nests they are building.)

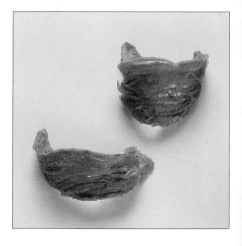

Nests are graded. The most expensive are white, whole, and very clean. Second-grade are pieces; lowest grade are cakes of compressed bits.

Gastronomically, bird's nest is a delicacy; medicinally, it is indicated chiefly in convalescence.

Cicada Molt *(Cryptotympana pustulata)* 蟬 蛻

[M] Chan tui; [C] Seem chuei

Action: Reduces persistent heat of fever; stops convulsions; eases skin eruptions, particularly in measles and chickenpox.

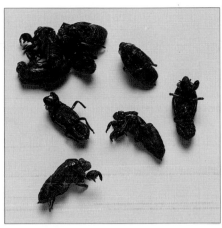

Use: Prescriptions.

Remarks: This is valued in children's prescriptions for its ability to control fever convulsions; similarly it stops convulsions in excessive cocaine use. It is also used in cases of persistent or recurrent fever as in malaria and in some cases of lung cancer.

Deer Antlers *(Cervi pantotrichum; Cervus nippon)* 鹿 茸

[M] Lu rong; [C] Look yoeng

Action: Invigorates the yang component of kidney energy; increases production of semen.

Use: Prescriptions; soups; wine infusions.

Remarks: This is arguably the most popular of the sexual tonics. In the Chinese medical system, kidneys control sexual function; hence, foods and herbs such as this which can invigorate the kidneys are used for impotence and infertility in both men and women.

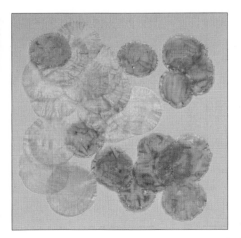

The best quality antlers are taken from young bucks, i.e., new horn still in velvet with blood visible in the cartilage. Whole antlers are extremely expensive; most customers buy fine slices which they then infuse in water or wine.

A
N
I
M
A
L

M
A
T
T
E
R

Donkey Hide Glue (*Equus asinau:* preparation) 阿膠

[M] E jiao; [C] Ngoh gau

Action: Tonifies the body by supplying energy; nourishes and invigorates yin; stimulates production of blood. [CR] Increases red blood cells, hemoglobin and blood platelets; promotes white blood cell (lymphocyte) transformation; balances calcium and clears deposits; prevents oxidation of vitamin E.

Use: Prescriptions; patent medicines.

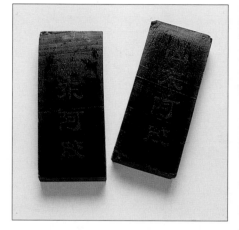

Remarks: This is prepared from the boiling of asses' hides. When used in prescriptions it is generally added last—after the other ingredients have been boiled. Its unusual ability to nourish the yin and the blood makes it a valuable universal tonic.

Praying Mantis Egg Case

(*Ootheca mantidis*) 桑螵蛸

[M] Sang piao xiao; [C] Song piu siu

Action: Invigorates the qi of the kidney; eliminates excess fluid from the body, i.e., can stop bleeding, excess perspiration, and leucorrhea.

Use: Prescriptions; patent medicines.

Remarks: This is a popular herb, especially among the elderly. As the kidney energy meridian nourishes the reproductive system, this herb is used for problems both of the kidney organ (e.g., incontinence) and of the male/female organs (e.g., nocturnal emission, leucorrhagia, impotence).

Seahorse *(Hippocampus kelloggii)* 海馬

[M] Hai ma; [C] Hoi ma

Action: Promotes kidney yang; normalizes sexual activity; good for the bones and the bone marrow.

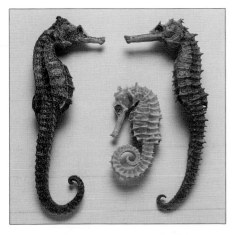

Use: Prescriptions; soups.

Remarks: When used in prescriptions, this is usually smashed or ground into powder. When used in soups, it is left whole. It is recommended for symptoms of weakness, dizziness and/or lethargy which are due to deficient yang, hence it is most commonly prescribed for the elderly. The white seahorses (center) have been bleached.

Turtle Shell *(Chinemys reevesii)* 龜板

[M] Gui ban; [C] Gwai baan

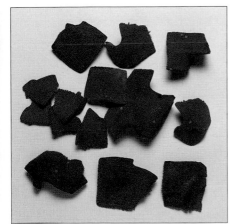

Action: Nourishes yin of liver, heart and kidneys; detoxifies the liver channel.

Use: Prescriptions; soups; desserts.

Remarks: The most conspicuous consumption of this herb is in the dessert "Gwai Ling Go", a black jelly made of turtle shell and China-root. It is available fresh at Cantonese herbal tea stores and packaged in supermarkets. It is considered to be a powerful detoxifier (for toxic symptoms ranging from acne to cancer) and nutrient for sinew and bone.

Gypsum *(Calcium sulfate)* 石膏

[M] Shi gao; [C] Sek go

Action: Drains fire from entire body; dries out the body and heals wounds due to wetness, e.g., boils, rashes.

Use: Prescriptions; soups.

Remarks: Medicinally, gypsum is used externally and internally. Externally, it is applied to skin abscesses which have not burst; it is added to soups and congee for, in particular, gum problems. Gypsum is even more valuable in the culinary sphere, as it is the traditional coagulating agent for beancurd. Much of the "sek go fun" bought by housewives is used to make a dessert known as "dao fu fa", similar to bean curd in its preparation and in taste and texture.

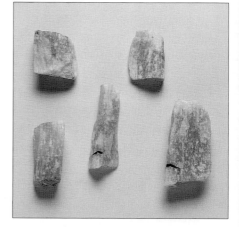

Pearl Dust *(Concha margaritifera usta)* 珍珠末

[M] Zhen zhu mu; [C] Jun ju moot

Action: Used internally, it detoxifies, especially clearing liver fire; stops convulsions. Used externally, stops ulcerations.

Use: Prescriptions; patent medicines.

Remarks: This is a traditional medicine which is being replaced by others. It is primarily used now to treat cataracts, which are considered to be a symptom of liver fire.

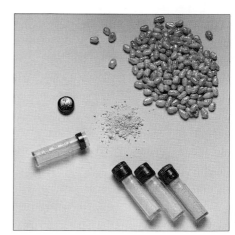

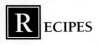

To the Chinese, and especially the Cantonese, soup is a vital element in the daily meal as a source of nourishment and as a means of maintaining health. Different soups are made according to the season (i.e., cooling soups in summer, warming soups in winter), or to help individuals with specific conditions, from arthritis and flu to stress at work.

Below are four of the most common and widely appropriate soups from this extensive repertoire.

CHING BO LEUNG 清補涼

This soup is a mild and general tonic, meant to be good for anyone in any condition. The ingredients—many of which target the cardiovascular system—help the body function properly without overstimulating any particular organ.

Premixed packets of the soup are sold in medicinal herb shops as well as grocery stores in Asian supermarkets. It is prepared both as a savory soup—typically using pork meat or bones for flavour—or as a sweet dessert soup, in which case sugar is added at the end.

Ingredients:

15 g pearl barley	薏米半兩
30 g polygonatum	玉竹一兩
30 g lotus seeds	蓮子一兩
30 g foxnuts	茨實一兩
15 g Chinese yam	淮山五錢
30 g lily bulbs	百合一兩
10 g dried longan (optional)	元肉或龍眼肉三錢
(Pork)	

Directions:

Combine all the ingredients in a large pot. Add approximately 8 cups of water—or enough to cover the ingredients by 3 times their volume—and pork meat or bones, if desired. Bring to the boil; reduce heat, and simmer partially covered until barley is cooked and liquid is reduced, 1-2 hours. Season with salt for a savory soup, or sweeten with sugar for a sweet soup.

HUI SUP LIU 去濕料

This soup regulates the water and electrolyte balance in the body. It is particularly appropriate in hot humid weather. Edema, fungal infections (e.g., athlete's foot) and red, puffy eyes are symptoms associated with a "wet" condition which would benefit from this "dampness-chasing" soup.

The following can be brewed alone or with winter melon and pork.

Ingredients:
20 g Job's tears barley	苡米七錢
30 g adzuki beans	赤小豆一兩
30 g hyacinth (lablab) beans	扁豆一兩
30 g tree cotton flowers	木棉花一兩
1 lotus seed pod	蓮房一個
(Winter melon)	冬瓜
(Pork)	

Directions:

If using the melon, wash it but do not peel or remove the seeds: chop coarsely, and add all into the soup pot. Combine everything; add water— approximately 8 cups or enough to cover the dry ingredients to 3 times their volume. Bring to the boil; reduce heat and simmer until beans and barley are cooked and liquid is reduced, at least one hour, preferably 2-3 if you are using meat. Season with salt and serve. (N.B. The melon, pork, beans and barley are edible, but not the kapok flower or lotus pod.)

KOREAN GINSENG CHICKEN SOUP 高麗參雞湯

This is a nourishing soup particularly beneficial for older people year-round and for anyone during the winter. As with "Ng Gwun Tong", those suffering from exopathic diseases (i.e., caused by forces external to the body, such as viral flu; not originating within the body, such as asthma) should avoid this lest the chicken and ginseng nourish their illness rather than them.

Ingredients:
   1 small chicken, about 500 g
   25 g Korean ginseng
   750 ml water

Combine ingredients in a non-metallic pot (earthenware is ideal), and simmer gently or double-boil for 4 hours. Season with salt if desired.

Ng Gwun Tong 五君湯

Like "Ching Bo Leung", this is a general tonic; however, this is more powerful in its action, and specifically not recommended for anyone suffering from externally-caused illness such as the flu. The particular ingredients comprising this soup are chosen to increase vital energy (qi) and to dredge the body's energy channels releasing blockages; as qi flows more vigorously and circulates freely it harmonizes the entire system.

Ingredients:		
	30 g dangshen	黨參一兩
	30 g milk vetch	黃芪一兩
	30 g Chinese yam	淮山一兩
	5 g wolfberry	枸杞子二錢
	6 g cordyceps or	冬蟲夏草二錢或
	9 g China-root	伏神三錢
	Chicken or lean pork	

Directions:

For boiling, combine ingredients in a large pot with water to a depth of approximately twice the volume of ingredients. Bring to the boil, reduce heat, and simmer partially covered until volume is reduced by half, 2-3 hours. Season to taste and serve.

For double-boiling, the ingredients and an equal volume of water are placed in a small, lidded, usually ceramic container within a larger pot. Water is added to the larger pot and brought to the boil. Ingredients in the inner container are hence cooked, but the lid retains subtle flavours otherwise lost when boiled directly. Double-boiling requires a minimum of 3-4 hours.

AMERICAN GINSENG TEA 花旗參茶

This is a popular infusion to boost flagging spirits, restore concentration, and revive the weary. Students take it during exams; mahjong players drink it as games stretch into the wee hours of the morning.

As in making tea, simply pour hot water over thin slices of the ginseng. Allow it to steep, then drink. Alternatively, you may put a few pieces in the bottom of a thermos, add hot water, and drink from there as required or desired. The flavor is strong; a few slices will indeed go a long way. When drinking this frequently, also add a small piece of licorice ([C] "gum cho" 甘草) to moisten the throat, which ginseng will tend to dry out.

CHRYSANTHEMUM TEA 菊花茶

Chrysanthemum is a sweeter, milder relative of chamomile; both are members of the sunflower plant family. Chrysanthemum flowers have properties which cleanse and cool the liver without, some Chinese herbalists say, interfering with the function of the stomach. Hence they are suitable for people of all ages, and can be enjoyed equally widely. Three styles of taking the tea are popular:

* The most simple preparation is to infuse the flowers alone as you would tea, using about a tablespoon of flowers per cup of boiling water. Allow to steep, and drink either hot or cold, plain or sweetened.

* Alternatively flowers may be added to regular tea. The Cantonese "gook-bo" refers to a combination of chrysanthemum flowers ("GOOK fa") with a particular red tea ("BO lei" 普洱). This is considered to be a perfectly balanced drink—both yin and yang are represented--and is available in many Cantonese restaurants.

* Chrysanthemum flowers may be boiled. In this case, they are usually combined in equal proportions with honeysuckle flowers (金銀花); add water, using approximately a tablespoon of flowers per cup; bring to the boil and then simmer until the liquid is well flavoured. Finally add rock sugar to taste as the brew will be bither.

English	Latin	Mandarin	Cantonese	Chinese	Page
Abalone	*Haliotis* spp.	Bao yu	Bao yu	鮑魚	42
Achyranthes	*Achyranthes bidentata*	Niu xi	Ngau chut	牛膝	16
Adzuki Beans	*Phaseolus calcaratus*	Chi xiao dou	Chek siu dau	赤小豆	31
Angelica	*Angelica sinensis*	Dang quai	Dong gwai	當歸	16
Apricot Kernels	*Prunus armeniaca*	Xing ren	Hung yun	杏仁	31
Baizhu	*Atractylodes macrocephala*	Bai zhu	Baak soot	白朮	17
Bird's Nest	*Collocalia* sp.: preparation	Yen wo	Yeen woh	燕窩	42
Cannabis (seeds)	*Cannabis sativa*	Huo ma ren	Foh ma yun	火麻仁	33
China-Root	*Poria cocos*	Fu ling	Fook ling	茯苓	17
Chinese Cornbind	*Polygonum multiflorum*	Shou wu	Sau wu	首烏	18
Chinese Foxglove	*Rehmannia glutinosa*	Di huang	Dei wong	地黃	18
Chinese Yam	*Dioscorea opposita*	Shan yao	Wai saan	山藥・淮山	19
Chrysanthemum (flowers)	*Chrysanthemum morifolium*	Ju hua	Gook fa	菊花	26
Cicada Molt	*Cryptotympana pustulata*	Chan tui	Seem chuei	蟬蛻	43
Cordyceps (Winter Worm-Summer Herb)	*Cordyceps sinensis*	Dong chong xia cao	Doeng choeng ha cho	冬蟲夏草	19
Corn Silk	*Zea mays*	Yu mi xu	Sook mai so	玉米鬚	26
Dandelion	*Taraxacum officinale*	Pu gong ying	Po gong ying	蒲公英	27
Dangshen	*Codonopsis* spp.	Dang shen	Dong sum	黨參	20
Dates	*Zizyphus jujuba*	Zao	Jo	棗	32
Dates , Black		Nan zao	Naam jo	南棗	32
Dates, Brown or Honey		Mi zao	Mut jo	蜜棗	32
Dates, Red		Hong zao	Hoeng jo	紅棗	32
Deer Antlers	*Cervi pantotrichum; Cervus nippon*	Lu rong	Look yoeng	鹿茸	43
Donkey Hide Glue	*Equus asinau:* preparation	E jiao	Ngoh gau	阿膠	44
Downy Artemesia	*Artemisia capillaris*	Yin chuen	Yan chun	茵陳	27
Ephedra	*Ephedra sinica*	Ma huang	Ma wong	麻黃	28
Eucommia	*Eucommia ulmoides*	Du zhong	Do joeng	杜仲	20
Fermented Black Soy Beans	*Glycine max:* preparation	Dan dou chi	Taam dau see	淡豆豉	33
Figs	*Ficus carica*	Wu hua guo	Mo fa gwoh	無花果	34
Forsythia	*Forsythia suspensa*	Lian qiao	Leen kiu	連翹	34
Foxnut	*Euryale ferox*	Qian shi	Chee sut	茨實	35
Ginger (dried)	*Zingiber officinale*	Gon jiang	Gon geung	乾薑	21
Ginkgo Nuts	*Ginkgo biloba*	Bai guo	Baak gwoh	白果	35
Ginseng, American	*Panax quinquefolium*	Yang shen	Fa kei sum	花旗參	12

English	Latin	Mandarin	Cantonese	Chinese	Page
Ginseng, Chinese or Korean	Panax ginseng	Gao li shen	Go lai sum	高麗參・人參	12
Ginseng, Russian or Siberian	Eleutherococcus senticosus	Chou shen	Chau sum	抽參	12
Golden Thread	Coptis chinensis	Huang lian	Wong leen	黃蓮	21
Gypsum	Calcium sulfate	Shi gao	Sek go	石膏	46
Hawthorn	Crataegus pinnatifida	Shan zha	Saan ja	山楂	36
Honeysuckle (flowers)	Lonicera japonica	Jin yin hua	Gum ngun fa	金銀花	28
Hyacinth Beans	Dolichos lablab	Bian dou	Been dau	扁豆	36
Job's Tears Barley	Coix lachryma-jobi	Yi yi ren	Yee mai	苡米仁・薏米	37
Licorice	Glycyrrhiza uralensis	Gan cao	Gum cho	甘草	22
Lily Bulbs	Lilium lancifolium	Bai he	Baat hup	百合	22
Lingzhi	Lucida ganoderma	Ling zhi	Ling ji	靈芝	37
Longan Fruit	Euphoria longan	Yun ron	Yoon yoek	圓肉	38
Loquat (leaves)	Eriobotrya japonica	Pi pa yeh	Pei pa yeep	枇杷葉	29
Lotus Seed Pods	Nelumbo nucifera	Lian fung	Leen fung	蓮房	38
Lotus Seeds	Nelumbo nucifera	Lian zi	Leen jee	蓮子	39
Mandarin Tangerine Peel	Citrus reticulata	Chen pi	Chun pei	陳皮	39
Milk Vetch	Astragalus spp.	Huang qi	Wong kei; but kei	黃芪・北芪	23
Mint	Mentha arvensis	Bo he	Bok haw	薄荷	29
Notoginseng	Panax notoginseng	San qi	Saam chut; teen chut	三七・田七	23
Peach Kernels	Prunus persisa	Tao ren	To yun	桃仁	40
Pearl Barley	Hordeum vulgare	Da mai	Yeung yee mai	大麥・洋苡米	40
Pearl Dust	Concha margaritifera usta	Zhen zhu mu	Jun ju moot	珍珠末	46
Peony	Paeonia moutan	Mu dan pi	Mao daan pei	牡丹皮	24
Polygonatum (Solomon's Seal)	Polygonatum odoratum	Yu zhu	Yook jook	玉竹	25
Praying Mantis Egg Case	Ootheca mantidis	Sang piao xiao	Song piu siu	桑螵蛸	44
Rhubarb	Rheum officinale	Da huang	Dai wong	大黃	24
Seahorse	Hippocampus kelloggii	Hai ma	Hoi ma	海馬	45
Self-Heal	Prunella vulgaris	Xia ku cao	Ha gu cho	夏枯草	30
Tree Cotton (flowers)	Bombax ceiba	Mu mien hua	Mook meen fa	木棉花	30
Turtle Shell	Chinemys reevesii	Gui ban	Gwai baan	龜板	45
Wheat	Triticum aestivum	Xiao mai	Siu mut	小麥	41
White Mulberry (branches)	Morus alba	Sang zhi	Song jee	桑枝	25
Wolfberry	Lycium chinense	Ji zi	Gau gei jee	枸杞子	41